Seybou Baba Diarra

Secondary acute intestinal intussusception in children

Seybou Baba Diarra

Secondary acute intestinal intussusception in children

in the pediatric surgery department of CHU Gabriel Touré

ScienciaScripts

Imprint

Cover image: www.ingimage.com

This book is a translation from the original published under ISBN 978-620-6-70252-8.

Publisher:
Sciencia Scripts
is a trademark of
Dodo Books Indian Ocean Ltd. and OmniScriptum S.R.L publishing group

120 High Road, East Finchley, London, N2 9ED, United Kingdom
Str. Armeneasca 28/1, office 1, Chisinau MD-2012, Republic of Moldova, Europe
Printed at: see last page
ISBN: 978-620-8-36033-7

Contents

DEDICACES

I give thanks to **Allah** the almighty, the clement and the merciful. Everything begins with him and everything ends with him. I thank him for giving me life, courage and health, without which this work would not have taken place.

To the Prophet Mohamed (pbuh): may the peace of God be upon him.

I dedicate this modest work to :

My father : Baba DIARRA

Dear Father, this work is yours. You believed in me and spared no effort to make me what I am today.

You guided me in my first steps, you taught me the meaning of honour, dignity, humility, morality, justice and forgiveness.

You were always a hard worker, rigorous and demanding of yourself and the whole family.

Please find in this work the expression of my deepest gratitude and of all my appreciation. Your prayers have never failed me, as have your encouragement and your moral, emotional and material support.

Thank you from the bottom of my heart because you have been the key to my success. May the Almighty Allah give you a long life with lots of health above all.

My mother : Djeneba COULIBALY

Dearest Mum, you embody for me the affection of a devoted, courageous and tolerant mother. Your love for us, your great generosity and your sense of forgiveness have always impressed me.

I'll never forget this maternal warmth and I'm at a loss for words to describe you and express all the love and admiration I have for you.

All the merit of this work is also yours. Thank you for your blessings, your daily prayers and all the sacrifices you have made for your children and your whole family.

May the Almighty Lord bless you and grant you a long life in peace and the greatest health.

To my horror: Aminata

You have been more than just a great sore thumb to me, as you have cultivated in me respect, honesty, courage and a sense of a job well done. This work would not have been possible without your efforts. I thought of you at every moment of this work.

My brothers and sisters: Bable, Salif, Mahamadou, Arouna and Mastan, Mariam, Kadidiatou, Alimata, Bintou

Dear brothers and sisters, thank you for your support, affection and respect for me. May the good Lord give me the courage to be grateful to you, and may he be the guarantor of our brotherhood.

My Aunts and Uncles : Awa DIARRA , Kadidiatou DIARRA, Wassa DIARRA, Mah DIARRA and Yacouba DIARRA, Adama DIARRA, Issa DIARRA, Soungo DIARRA

My dear aunts and uncles, thank you for your advice and affection for me.

ACKNOWLEDGEMENTS

Glory be to God, creator of the heavens and the earth, the omniscient and omnipotent. It is to you that we seek refuge and it is to you that we ask for wisdom, for we have no knowledge other than what you have taught us. We thank the Prophet Muhammad (SAW) for the good news; we will be faithful to you until our last breath. May your family and all those who follow you enter paradise.

My sincerest thanks go to:

To the COULIBALY family, my thanks, respects and considerations.

To Dr Mamadou TRAORE, I can't thank you enough.

To all the staff at CHU - Gabriel TOURE for your availability.

To all my comrades and friends at Point-G, with whom I went through all the difficult times.

To the Dean's Office and the teaching staff of the Faculty of the FMOS: who were kind enough to teach me and share their immense knowledge with me.

To all those, far or near, who have contributed to my training or to the preparation of this work.

To all those who show contempt for me.

To my master trainers:

Pr KEITA Mamby, Pr COULIBALY Yacaria, Dr TOURE Issa Amadou, Dr COULIBALY Oumar, Dr KAMATE Benoi, Dr DOUMBIA Aliou, Dr DJIRE Mohamed Khassoum, Dr DAOU Moussa.

You've been more than teachers to me, so I hope you'll find in this document the fruit of your own efforts.

To Dr COULIBALY Youssouf, who has helped me so much throughout this work, you have been an unfailing support in the preparation of this document.

You remain a man concerned about the success of your young brothers. You have my sincere gratitude.

To the entire 9eme class of the FMOS numerus clausus, the late Pr ALWATA, in memory of the good times we had together.

To my friends in paediatric surgery:

Dr MAIGA Moussa, Dr TOGOLA Boubacar, Dr KONE Amadou, Dr KONTA Gaoussou, Dr HAIDARA Mahamadou, Dr DIARRA Drissa, Dr CAMARA Sadio, Dr COULIBALY Moussa, Dr SIDIBE Modibo, Dr BAH Mamadou Aliou.

Thank you for your advice and moral support.

Interns in paediatric surgery:

SAMAKE Ibrahima, TOGO Yacouba, SANGARE Sidiki, KEITA Victor,

DEMBELE Sekou, TRAORE Abdoul Kader, DIARRA Adama, TAPILY Aboubakar, SYLLA Salim, DIARRA Helene, TRAORE Fanta, AREMU Issuf, DIALLO Moussa O, DIALLO Mohamed S, NIARE Mamadou, COULIBALY Mariam, BAH Sekou, TRAORE Moustapha.

I had an unforgettable time with you and good luck on the job market.

To my cadets in paediatric surgery:

NIARE Daouda, DIALLO Lanseni, SIMAGA Oumar, COULIBALY Mamadou, GOITA Sidi, KEITA Naremba, BAH Kadidiatou, BERTHE Habibatou

I wish you courage and all the best for the future.

To all the nursing staff on the ward, Major Abdrahamane and his team: Koromba, Ouley, Djelika, Mme DIARRA, DOLO, SOUSSABA, Mariam dite Marie, AWA and all the others.

Thank you for your cooperation.

To my friends and confidants: THIOCARY Sinaly, TRAORE Arouna, TRAORE Mamadou, DENA Thomas

Thank you for your confidence in me; I'll never forget it.

TRIBUTE TO THE MEMBERS OF THE JURY

To our Master and President of the jury

Professor Alhassane TRAORE

- Associate Professor of General Surgery at the FMOS.
- Hospital practitioner at CHU Gabriel Toure.
- Specialist in hepatobiliary and pancreatic surgery.
- Lecturer at the Institut National de Formation en Science de la Sante
- Member of the Societe de Chirurgie du Mali (SO.CHI.MA).
- Member of 1 Association des Chirurgiens d'Afrique Francophone (A.C.A.F).
- Member of the International Hernia Society.

Dear Master,

You are doing us a great honour by agreeing to chair this jury, despite your many important commitments.

Your approachability, your critical mind and your scientific rigour make you a master respected and admired by all.

Please accept, dear master, the expression of our deep gratitude and unfailing attachment.

To our Master and Judge

Dr Belco MAIGA

> Assistant Master at the FMOS
> Hospital practitioner at CHU-Gabriel Toure
> Head of the paediatric emergency and intensive care unit at the Gabriel Toure University Hospital

Dear Master,

You have done us a great honour by agreeing to sit on this jury despite your many commitments. We were impressed by your modesty, your availability and your rigour in a job well done. Rest assured, dear Master, of our deep gratitude.

To our Master and co-director

Dr Issa AMADOU

> Assistant Professor of Paediatric Surgery at the FMOS
> Specialist in paediatric orthopaedics and traumatology
> Hospital practitioner at CHU Gabriel TOURE
> Membra de la SOCHMA
> Membra of AMAPED
> Membra of the African Society of Paediatric Surgeons

Dear Master,

You have always responded favourably to our work-related requests. Your presence is an opportunity for us to express our admiration for your professional competence and your great sympathy. You have our deepest gratitude.

To our Master and Director of These

Professor Yacaria COULIBALY

> Associate Professor of Paediatric Surgery at the FMOS
> Member of the Mali Surgical Society
> Hospital practitioner at CHU Gabriel TOURE
> Member of the African Society of Paediatric Surgeons
> Member of the Malian Association of Paediatrics
> Chevalier de l'ordre de merite de la sante

Dear Master,

You welcomed us into your department and shared your knowledge with us, demonstrating your commitment to our training. We would like to take this opportunity to thank you sincerely. Your frankness, your intellectual capacity and your rigour in a job well done are admired by all. Please accept, dear master, the expression of our deepest gratitude. You have our deepest respect.

1 INTRODUCTION

Intestinal invaginationtiiguc[1] (IIA) is the penetration of an intestinal segment and its meso into the underlying intestinal segment, by a mechanism of overturning in a finger of glove [1, 2, 3].

It is said to be secondary (IIAS) when it is linked to an organic lesion (Meckel's diverticulum, benign or malignant tumour) or is part of a more general pathology of the digestive tract (rheumatoid purpura, cystic fibrosis, celiac disease), or occurs in a particular context (postoperative IIA, chemotherapy, parasitosis). It is a rare abdominal emergency [4].

It is seen in newborns, infants under 2 months and children over 2 years of age, and accounts for 2.5% to 18% of IIA in children [4].

In Europe, recent studies estimate the rate at between 0.66 and 2.2 per 1000 children [5].

AKBULUT [6] in 2012 published a series of 36 cases of intestinal intussusception secondary to lymphoma.

The etiology was post-operative in the ONGOM series [7] in Uganda, which reported 37 cases in 2012.

In 2016, ENEHWI in Marrakech recorded 13 cases of IIA following Meckel's diverticulum [8].13 cases reported by MHANNA in 2015 had multiple causes [9].

In Mali in 2012, it accounted for 10.1% of acute intestinal obstructions [10].

It is predominant in gargons [3].

The diagnosis of IIA in children is easy, when the symptomatology is obvious and consists of the classic triad of paroxysmal abdominal pain, vomiting and rectal discharge. However, this triad is not always present, as the symptomatology may be atypical, confusing the practitioner and delaying management [11].

The difficulty in diagnosing ISAI lies in the diversity of incomplete or misleading clinical forms. It is generally suggested because of the age of onset, associated symptoms, location or recurrent nature of the intussusception.

Treatment is exclusively surgical and adapted to the etiology [3].

The prognosis depends on the duration of the disease, the extent of the lesions and the nature of the cause [3].

In order to compensate for the lack of data on IIAS in our department and to contribute to the development of the literature on this subject, we initiated this work, which had the following objectives.

2 OBJECTIVES

OBJECTIVES :

1- General objective :

Study of secondary acute intestinal intussusception in children in the paediatric surgery department of the CHU Gabriel Toure.

2- Specific objectives :

- Determining the hospital frequency of secondary acute intestinal intussusception in children;
- Determining the causes of secondary acute intestinal intussusception in children.
- Diagnostic and therapeutic aspects;
- Analysing the follow-up to the treatment.

3 GENERAL INFORMATION

GENERAL:

1- HISTORY:

Acute intestinal intussusception was distinguished from other intestinal obstructions less than 300 years ago. It was known before the advent of radiology, but its clinical diagnosis was often delayed.

John HUNTER (1793) described the acute invagination[1] and discussed its pathological anatomy post mortem.

In 1831, in Tennessee, WILSON performed the first surgical disinvagination on a black slave.

In 1871, Jonathan HUTCHINSON reported the first case to be successfully treated surgically.

In 1897, CLUBBE in Australia carried out the first invagination resection.

The first anatomical description of acute intussusception[1] is attributed to Paul Barbette in 1674 [12]. In the 19th century, some successful treatments using hydrostatic reduction were described, but the condition was usually fatal. The first curative procedure was performed in 1871 by Jonathan Hutchinson [13]. The diagnostic and therapeutic use of opaque enema was reported in 1927, in France by Pouliquen, in the United States by Retan and Stephens and in Scandinavia by Olsson and Pallin[14].

At the same time, the mortality rate for this condition fell from 75% in 1884 [19] to 30% in 1939 [15]. Since 1970, the mortality rate has been close to 0% [16].

2- DEFINITION:

Acute intestinal intussusception[1] (IIA) in children is the penetration of an intestinal segment and its mesentery into the segment immediately downstream, and its progression in an iso peristaltic direction in a person aged 15 or under.

The combination of the internal or invaginated cylinder, the external or invaginating cylinder and the intermediate cylinder(s) is known as the invaginated bladder. The result is a stoppage of intestinal transit responsible for a cessation of matter and gas, accompanied by venous compression with redema and hydrolytic disorders that can rapidly progress to intestinal necrosis. It is a medical and surgical emergency [1, 2, 3].

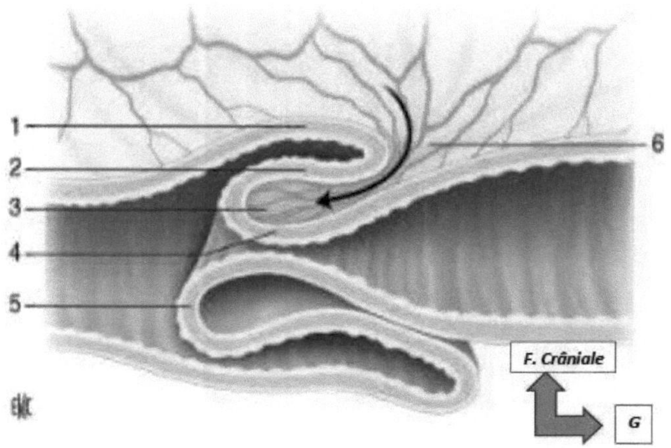

Figure 1: Invagination diagram
1= External tunic, 2= Middle tunic or return segment, 3= Meso-invagina, 4= Internal tunic or penetrating segment, 5= Head and 6= Collar. [3]

3- EPIDEMIOLOGY:

Secondary IIA is a rare abdominal surgical emergency.

It accounts for 2.5 to 18% of IIA. Its frequency is higher in series where surgery is systematic [4].

Sex distribution: secondary acute intussusception is predominantly male, with a sex ratio of 3 gargons to 2 girls [4].

Breakdown by age :

Secondary lIA in children typically occurs between the ages of 2 months and over 2 years [17, 18].

4- ANATOMOPATHOLOGY:

Invaginations are referred to firstly by the name of the invaginated intestinal segment, then by the name of the intermediate intestinal segment that may have been involved, and finally by the name of the invaginated segment. Iliocolic intussusception is the most common; it starts in the terminal ileum, then spreads through the colon to a greater or lesser extent towards the anus, which it may reach. The intussusception is said to be ileocolicTrans valvular when Bauhin's valve and the appendix remain in place. It is ileo-coeco-colic when the Bauhin valve forms the head of the intussusception, dragging the appendix into the intussusception process. Pure ileo-ileal or pure colo-colic intussusception are rare variants of idiopathic intussusception. The simplest intussusception consists of three cylinders.

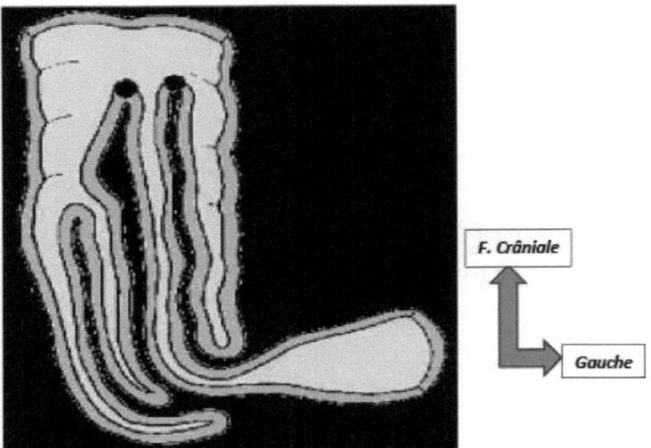

Figure 2: Ileo-caeco-colic invagination

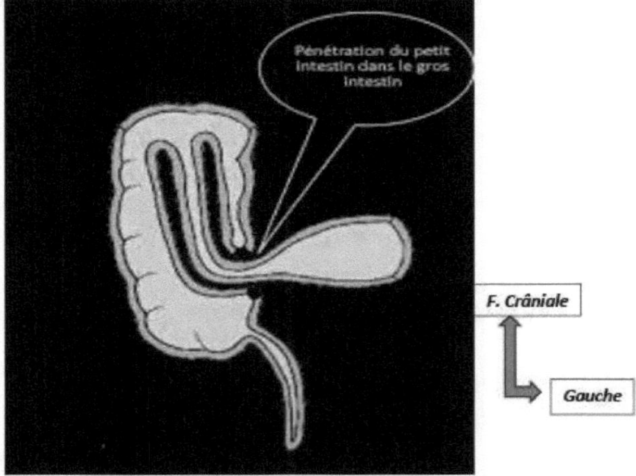

Figure 3: Transvalvular ileocolic invagination

Depending on the topography, a distinction is made between :

- acute intestinal intussusception with an ileo-caecal origin (90% of cases): - ileo-caecal - C®co-c®cales - Ileo-colics
- tiiguc's intestinal invaginations with an ileal starting point: - Ileo-ileals by mechanical obstruction - Ileo-colics - Ileo-c®cales
- intestinal invaginations tiiguc's with a colonic starting point :
- Right colon, more common in older children

- Colo-colic intussusception:

It is inconstantly secondary and rare in children (polyp, duplication).

5- ETIOLOGY:

In general, IIAS is associated with intestinal motor disorders, the causes of which are now very diverse.

In infants, the density of Payer plaques and mesenteric lymph nodes in the ileo-caecal region is very high.

The male predominance of IIA is explained by the greater lymphoid tissue in the gargon than in the girl.

A distinction is made between intussusceptions secondary to so-called organic lesions, which are more common in children or associated with another pathology, and so-called idiopathic intussusceptions, which represent the majority of cases (90% in infants).

Parietal lesions (Meckel's diverticulum, duplication, polyp, benign or malignant tumour, gastrointestinal stromal tumour, inflammatory pseudotumour) or a general disease of the digestive tract (lymphoma, rheumatoid purpura, cystic fibrosis, celiac disease) can also constitute an obstacle to intestinal motricity and are responsible for secondary intussusception.

Some authors report a hereditary predisposition, which may be considered as an etiology of IIA, especially after a viral infection [19].

There is also postoperative IIA, which is exclusive to children and occurs in the days following surgery that modifies the intestinal and especially mesenteric topography (especially the retroperitoneum, exeresis of a large mass) [20, 21, 22].

6- PATHOPHYSIOLOGY:

1. Mechanisms :

In the majority of cases (98%), IIA is linked to a disorder of intestinal peristalsis.

The hypertrophy of the lymphoid tissue, which is very important in infants in the ileo-c®cal region, constitutes the starting point for intussusception, creating an obstacle to intestinal peristalsis, which is sometimes increased by viral infection (there are usual seasonal peaks, and epidemics have even been reported, probably related to the existence of a viral infection). The peristaltic wave from one intestinal segment does not propagate and collides with the underlying relaxed segment, causing it to overturn [1].

An association between the use of antibiotics and the occurrence of AII has been identified, as antibiotics are the most frequently prescribed drugs in the paediatric population. Moreover, they have adverse effects on the gastrointestinal tract by modifying the motricity of the intestinal flora [3].

Parietal lesions (Meckel's diverticulum, duplication, gall bladder polyp, hemangioma or other benign or malignant tumour) or a more general disease of

the digestive tract (lymphoma, rheumatoid purpura) may also constitute etiologies of intestinal intussusception [4].
Hemolytic uremic syndrome (HUS) leads to intestinal vascular disorders and is responsible for abnormalities in the viscosity of intestinal contents. These lesions can lead to so-called secondary acute intestinal invaginations [23].
Postoperative IIA is a classic but rare complication of abdominal surgery. Rare in adults, it is the consequence in children of alterations in intestinal motor function in the postoperative phase due to multiple pre-, per- and postoperative factors [22].
Several favourable factors have been noted in cases of IIA following abdominal neuroblastoma surgery: the child's young age, preoperative anticancer chemotherapy, prolonged general anaesthesia and long dissection of the retroperitoneum in contact with the nervous elements of the neurovegetative system [24].
Chemotherapy is a rarer cause in children treated for malignant tumours; thickening of the intestinal walls is responsible for hyperperistalsis leading to intestinal invagination [25].
Exclusive breastfeeding may also be a risk factor for IIA, through increased intestinal peristalsis [1].
Spontaneous disinvagination is also possible, and this explains the painful attacks suggestive of IIA sometimes found in patients' antecedents.

2. Consequences :

- The local consequences of acute intussusception are twofold:

1. Occlusion by obstruction of the intestinal lumen, resulting in strangulation of the mesentery of the invaginated segment, which is what makes the disease so serious.
2. The venous and lymphatic compression resulting from this strangulation is responsible for both redeme and mucosal hypersecretion.

In more advanced forms, fluid stasis can be observed upstream of the boudin, with the formation of a veritable 3rd intestinal sector enhanced by extravasation of intra-peritoneal fluid. Compression of the nervous elements explains the neurovegetative reactions accompanying attacks of heat, and mesenteric arterial compression leads to ischaemia and then necrosis of the wall of the intussusception loop, with diffusion of blood into the digestive tract.

- The General Consequences are linked to:

❖ Local factors:

S Hydrolytic imbalance, leading to acute dehydration.

S Acid-base balance.

S Hemodynamic imbalance is due to hypovolemia secondary to the 3rd sector and dehydration.

S Ventilatory repercussions are responsible for abdominal distension, which leads to alveolar hypoventilation.

S Toxi-infectious state: by intra-peritoneal dissemination of intestinal germs.

S Neurovegetative reactions: by compression of nerve elements.

Type of description: IIA secondary to Meckel's diverticulum (DM)

It is rare, occurring in only 2% of individuals. It is always single, implanted opposite the termination of the superior mesenteric artery. It is vascularised by a separate arterial branch arising from the arcade bourdante [26, 27].

Usually latent, it can be discovered by chance. However, it can give rise to certain complications, particularly in children, especially if they are young: 30% of complications before the age of 1, 40% before the age of 10.

Although the distribution of Meckel's diverticulum is approximately equal between the sexes. These complications have a very clear male predominance, between 70 and 90% for the majority of authors.

Intestinal obstruction is the most serious and most frequent form of Meckel's diverticulum, and occurs mainly in infants and children.

The most common mechanism is tiiguc intestinal intussusception[1] (more rarely, a volvulus, a flange or a kink is the cause of the obstruction). This usually occurs in older children over the age of 2 years [28, 29].

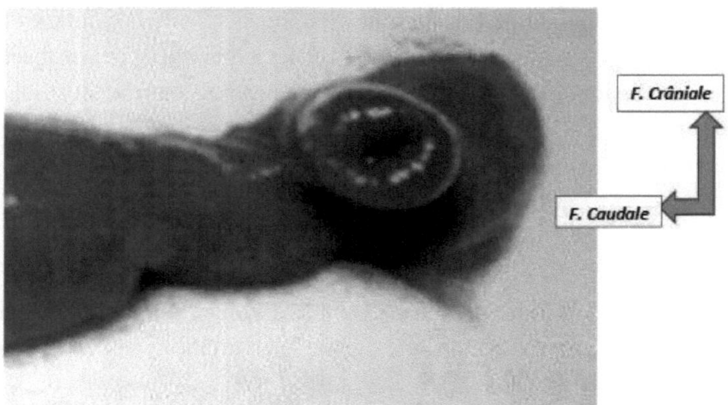

Figure 4: Invaginated Meckel diverticulum

o Functional sign:

a. Paroxysmal pain attacks :

- Pain is most often the main symptom. It is evocative when it occurs in paroxysmal episodes separated by free intervals.
- It may wake the child at night. It brings a sudden halt to activity, with the child screaming and folding his legs. Subsequent attacks follow each other with

varying frequency.

- In 15% of cases, the pain is unspecific, making diagnosis more difficult [30, 31].

b. vomiting

- Vomiting of food often accompanies the first attack, but is not constant during subsequent attacks. On the other hand, in infants, bottle refusal is almost constant, and is therefore a good sign in favour of this diagnosis.
- Bilious vomiting generally points towards a form seen late (at the stage of intestinal obstruction) or a particular anatomical form (upper ileo-ileal or jejuno-jejunal intussusception) [1].

c. Rectorrhagia :

- Early on, these are red or black bloody streaks, originating from the ischemic mucosa. They have no prognostic value. However, when bleeding is observed outside the first attack, this indicates extensive parietal damage and should raise the suspicion of intestinal necrosis [2].

3. Occlusive syndrome :

- The cessation of fluid and gas is often observed in late-onset forms. However, it is important not to wait until this triad is complete before carrying out the paraclinical tests that will confirm the diagnosis, as each of the symptoms can often appear in isolation.
- Transit can be maintained during the first attacks. This is a reflex emptying of the downstream intestine. Transit then ceases completely or, in the event of incomplete occlusion, persists in the form of misleading diarrhoeal stools.

o General signs:

Fever, asthenia, heat, dehydration, adynamia, even coma, sometimes a state of shock.

o Physical signs:

1. Inspection:

A quick inspection will reveal the extent to which the intussusception has affected the child's general condition: signs of dehydration, asthenia, hypotonia, heat, etc.

Inspection of the abdomen can reveal abdominal meteorism or localized bloating in relation to a gallbladder obstruction.

2. Abdominal palpation:

Abdominal palpation should be performed carefully, with warm hands, outside of painful attacks. The right iliac fossa appears to be classically uninhabited and easily depressed, localising the sign of

DANCE. It is sometimes in the right hypochondrium that palpation causes pain and reveals the intussusception bulge in the form of a firm, elongated, cylindrical and mobile mass. This bulge should be sought along the entire length of the colonic frame. Check that the hernial orifices are empty; palpation will look for the bulge, often in vain.

However, heavy weather can also make it difficult to palpate the bladder.

3. Percussion:

Tympany can sometimes be found.

4. Abdominal auscultation:

Hydro-aerobic sounds normal or absent in the case of necrosis.

5. Rectal examination:

Although not systematic, it can provide an additional sign in favour of the diagnosis. Very rarely, it may be possible to see the head of the pudding when it has made its way into the rectal ampulla or caused bloody stools to be passed.

- o Paraclinical signs:

1. The unprepared abdomen:

Typical signs of intussusception are :

- a tissue image reminiscent of a sausage;
- a "target" image consisting of a ring of fat density surrounding a water opacity containing a fat centre;
- a "crescent" image of the head of the bladder silhouetted by the air of the downstream digestive segment.

The following may also be involved:

- signs of graft occlusion or, on the contrary, poor digestive aeration;
- the absence of calcareous granite, with the coves being drawn towards the right iliac fossa (FID).
- In this case, the unprepared abdomen, taken from the front and standing upright, shows water-aerated levels on the body.

The PSA should look for an exceptional pneumoperitoneum, which would contraindicate any diagnostic or therapeutic enema.

This examination is only useful for demonstrating certain complications of Meckel's diverticulum, such as occlusion [1].

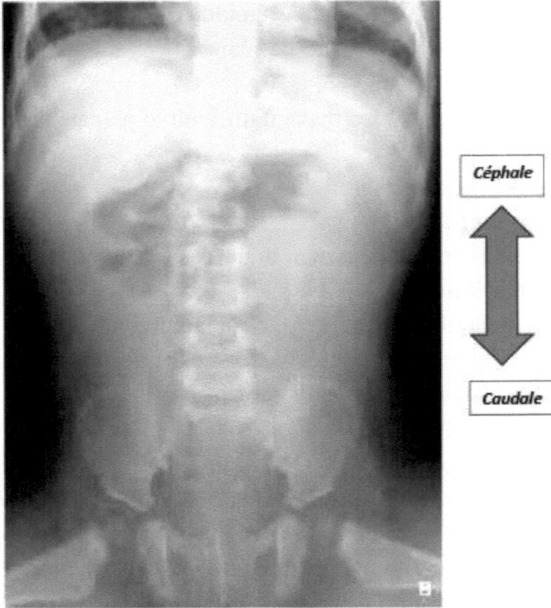

Figure 5: ASP, showing occlusion of the gracle

2. Abdominal ultrasound :

It is the key diagnostic test, with a sensitivity and negative predictive value close to 100%. It is carried out on a calm child, enabling the entire abdomen and digestive structures to be examined. All areas of the abdomen should be explored, and the head of the intussusception coil may extend as far as the rectum [32, 33].

The ileocolic or colocolic intussusception bulge measures between 3 and 5 cm in diameter and is located under the abdominal wall. It is therefore an "easy" mass to detect on ultrasound. Greco-colic intussusceptions have the same characteristics as ileo-colic intussusceptions.

semiology, but their diameter is less than 3 cm. they tend to be located centrally or in the left flank, and are sometimes more difficult to detect.

The characteristic images are :

> In transverse section, the "cocarde" image, made up of a rather hyperechogenic peripheral crown made up of several digestive layers and including an eccentric hyperechogenic crescent, can be seen.

corresponding to the mesentere incarcere.

> In longitudinal section, the so-called "sandwich" or "pseudo-rein" image corresponds to the succession of layers of hypoechogenic digestive wall in

relation to the more central, hyperechogenic mesenteric fat. The area of penetration of the invaginated loop into the receiving loop can be perfectly visualised. The vascular pedicle is also visible on colour Doppler.

Ultrasound can also be used to diagnose secondary forms, such as Meckel's diverticulum, digestive duplication or lymphoma. It can also be used to make a differential diagnosis with other causes of abdominal pain: mesenteric adenitis, volvulus, appendicitis.

It also enables complications to be detected:

> Occlusion (detected before the standard click).

> Peritoneal effusion.

> Intestinal ischaemia: in very tight forms of acute intestinal invagination[1] , with incipient vascular damage, particularly in ileo-ileal or ileo-colonic forms. There is often an effusion of fluid between the layers of the invaginated segment, giving an anechoic crescent-shaped image. A lack of vascularity on Doppler examination, particularly in the head of the sulcus, is considered by some authors to be a sign of ischaemia, and is therefore contraindicative of any attempt at reduction.

> Perforation: more or less echogenic intra-peritoneal effusion, extra-intestinal gas.

NB: The ultrasound diagnosis of Meckel's diverticulum is exceptional. It is described as a blind digestive structure with a thick and differentiated wall, of variable rounded morphology "Digestive target image".

It sometimes reveals a mass with a hyperechogenic centre and a hypoechogenic peripheral ring, which may correspond to an inverse Meckel's diverticulum.

o Ultrasound can also be used to suggest surgery in 10% of cases, in the presence of complicated forms, secondary forms and forms showing a fluid crescent within the sulcus (Figure 6).

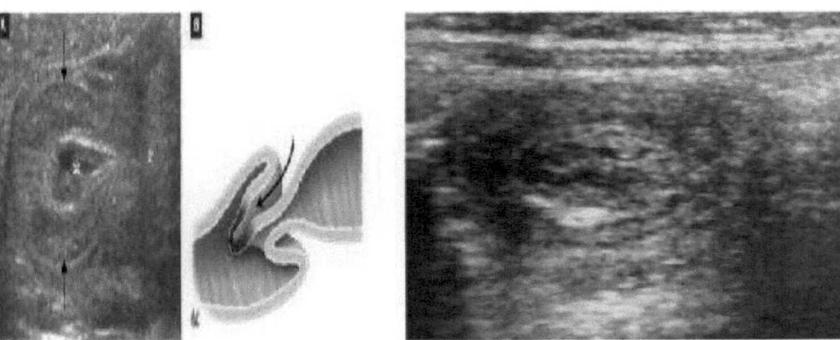

Figure 6:

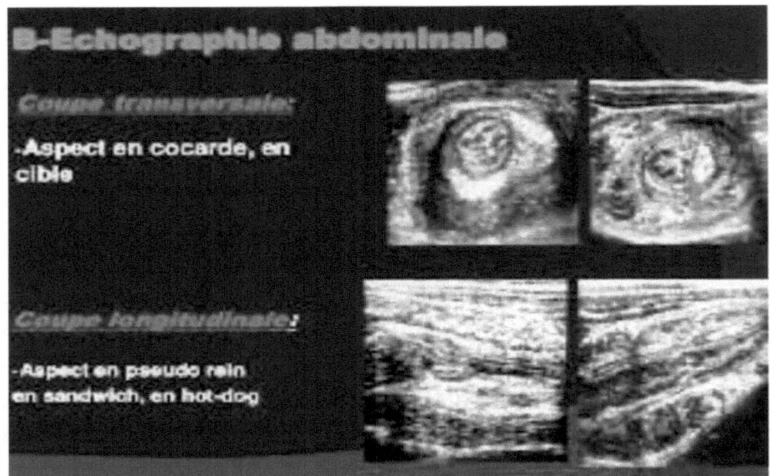

Figure 7: Cross-sections and longitudinal sections (cockade and sandwich appearance)

3- Hydrostatic or pneumatic enema:

In the presence of an experienced radiologist, the first-line use of enema to diagnose intussusception is no longer justified, as it has a negative effect in over 50% of cases.

The characteristic appearance is that the opaque or aerial column stops progressing at the level of the flange, giving it a lobster claw appearance.

On a barium enema, or on a transit of the grele: the topography of intraluminal lesions (polyposis).

At present, therefore, ultrasound is of no use in diagnosing secondary intestinal intussusception.

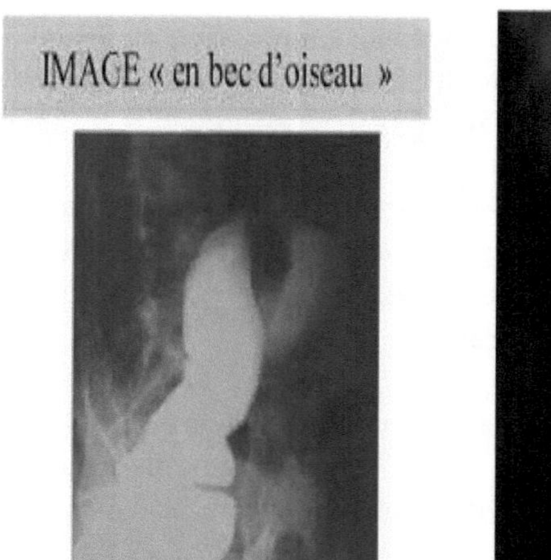

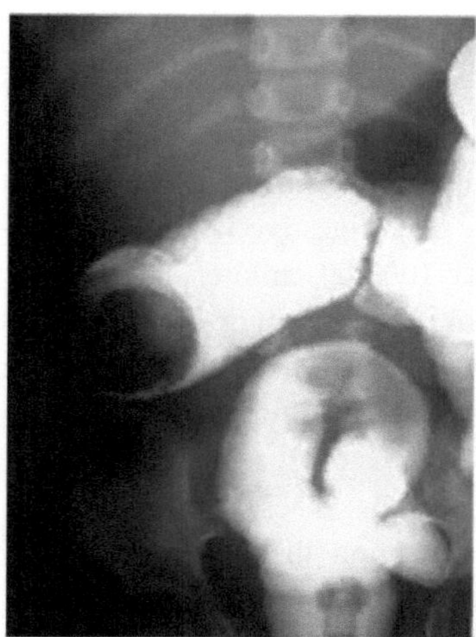

Figure 8: ***Cup stop*** ***Figure 9:***

4. Abdominal scan:

Widely indicated in adults, its use in children is limited to cases of secondary intussusception without evidence of a local cause on abdominal ultrasound.

It enables a positive diagnosis of invagination to be made and the causative lesion to be described (site, spontaneous density and after injection of contrast medium, relationship to neighbouring structures).

Abdominal CT scan: visible soft tissue invagination or mass.

The site of the invagination, the local cause: its density and enhancement.

The presence of an effusion.

5. Biology :

It enables the impact of secondary IIA to be assessed (CBC, blood ionogram, preoperative work-up).

CLINICAL FORMS:

1. Neonatal forms

Intussusception of the newborn is rare, and is usually induced by the presence of an intestinal malformation (cystic duplication of the cecum). The presence of rectal discharge or palpation of a sulcus is diagnostic, and the diagnosis is most often made preoperatively. This condition has been described in premature infants, where the clinical presentation frequently mimics ulcerative enterocolitis [1].

2. Tumours of the digestive tract

a. Intestinal polyps :

Lipoma is the 2nd most common benign tumour after adenoma. It accounts for 10% of benign tumours of the digestive tract and 2 to 4% of benign colonic tumours. Intestinal lipoma is rarely discovered by invagination. It is most often found in the cecum or ascending colon, and much more rarely in the left colon. In exceptional cases, the lipoma is responsible for intussusception. This risk appears from a diameter of 3cm [34, 35].

b. Digestive lymphomas:

It may be a digestive lymphoma, the incidence of which in western countries is 0.2 per 100,000 children under the age of 16 per year. Diagnosis is made by puncture of the mass or cytology of the ascites fluid [36, 37, 38, 39, 40].

3. Malformations of the digestive tract :

a. Digestive duplications :

Duplications of the ileo-c®cal junction are rare, and are most frequently incriminated. These malformations most often result in an ileo-ileal intussusception that is not visible with a barium enema, and is difficult to diagnose by ultrasound [41, 42].

b. Tissue heterotopy :

These lesions usually lead to ileo-ileal intussusception, which is not visible on a barium enema and is difficult to diagnose by ultrasound.

If there is clinical evidence of this, the patient should be referred for surgery [43].

C. Post-operative intestinal intussusception

It is defined as an intussusception that occurs after abdominal surgery other than intussusception surgery. It also occurs during the operative phase. The clinical signs vary and include bilious vomiting, an increase in the amount of digestive fluid collected by the gastric tube, abdominal distension, intermittent pain and rectal bleeding [20, 21, 22].

D. Rheumatoid purpura

IIA is a classic complication of rheumatoid purpura. It is diagnosed in 3-10% of cases, and most often during the course of overt rheumatoid purpura.

Diagnosis is difficult because abdominal pain, vomiting and rectal bleeding are all part of the purpura picture, which is linked to a diffuse vasculitis responsible for redness and bleeding of the digestive wall [44]. In two-thirds of cases, the II is ileo-isolated and therefore inaccessible to radiological reduction [45].

Treatment is often surgical, and the indication for surgery is difficult to establish. It should be guided by the clinical, radiological and ultrasound evolution, as it determines the prognosis in the acute phase [46, 47].

E. Cystic fibrosis

Cystic fibrosis is linked to the impact of mucus and occurs in less than 1% of cases. It occurs at an earlier age, between 9 and 12 years [48].

Along with ileus, caused by the impaction of very adherent material into the cecum in large children, it is one of the causes of abdominal pain and occlusion [49, 50].

This is an excellent indication for ultrasound examination. The opaque enema should be taken with a hyperosmolar water-soluble product in a rehydrated child. Early diagnosis increases the chances of hydrostatic reduction of the intussusception and allows evacuation of the faeces, thus avoiding surgery in these patients [1].

F. Chemotherapy

Methotrexate has been implicated because children can develop dysperistalsis and thickening of the intestinal walls, which favours the onset of IIA, which is usually ileo-iliac. Diagnosis is often delayed due to the subacute nature of the clinical manifestations. Ultrasound examination may be decisive if there is any doubt [24, 25].

G. Rare causes :

> **Celiac disease :**

The association of acute intestinal intussusception and celiac disease has been described since 1969 in adults and adolescents. Its description in children is more recent. The mechanism of these intussusceptions specific to celiac disease has not been fully elucidated [51].

> **Parasitic etiologies :**

Intestinal invagination of parasitic origin is rare, although a few cases have been reported in which trichocephalus has been identified in the form of adult glasses [52, 53].

> **Other causes include intestinal tuberculosis [54, 55] and Bezoard [56, 57].**

Anatomical shapes

The naming of intestinal invaginations uses first the name of the invaginated intestinal segment, then the name of the intermediate intestinal segment that may have been involved, and finally the name of the invaginated segment [58].

1. Ileo-iliac intussusception:

This is the most common form of secondary intestinal intussusception. It is most often secondary to parietal lesions (Meckel's diverticulum, duplication, polyp, angioma, hematoma, etc.) or any other tumour, whether isolated or linked to a general disease (lymphoma, rheumatoid purpura, etc.).

In this form, the head of the coil and its collar are formed by the ileon.

As they progress, they may cross Bauhin's valve, creating an ileo-ileo-transvalvular invagination, the ileo-ileal component of which may be detected during hydrostatic reduction [44].

2. Intussusception of the colon:

This is the most common form of idiopathic IIA. It starts in the terminal ileum and then spreads into the colon, sometimes reaching as far as the anus. Invagination is termed transvalvular ileocolic when Bauhin's valve and the appendix remain in place [Figure 3], and ileocolic when the appendix is invaginated and Bauhin's valve is at the apex of the bladder [Figure 2].

3. Colo-colic intussusception :

It is inconstantly secondary and rare in children (polyp, duplication).

4. Invagination of the appendix :

It's an exceptional form.

7- DIAGNOSTIC

1. Positive diagnosis :

The clinical diagnosis of IIAS is based on the classic triad of revealing signs: paroxysmal attacks of pain, vomiting and rectal bleeding. It is confirmed by an unprepared abdominal X-ray, abdominal ultrasound or abdominal CT scan.

2. Differential diagnosis :

- Primary acute intestinal invagination[1] (Idiopathic),

-Peritonitis: Contracture, fever, PSA and ultrasound help to correct the diagnosis.

- Acute appendicitis[1] : clinical and ultrasound diagnosis.
- Mesenteric adenolymphitis: clinical and ultrasound diagnosis.
- Gastroenteritis: clinical and ultrasound diagnosis.

Other causes of acute intestinal obstruction[1] : volvulus, bridges, tumours. Abdominal ultrasound and PSA confirm the diagnosis.

8- TREATMENT

1. Preventive treatment:

Minimise the need for surgery, by carrying out a good history-taking and clinical examination. This will enable us to reduce postoperative invaginations and even white laparotomy.

2- Curative treatment :

Surgical treatment is indicated whenever secondary intestinal intussusception is suspected. Surgery is performed as a matter of course to treat the organic lesion at the start of the intussusception, but also for fear of allowing a malignant tumour to develop.

2-1. Goal:

- Restore normal intestinal transit.
- Treat the possible cause.
- Preventing complications

2-2. Methods and resources :

2-2-1 Medical methods and resources :

This involves pre-, per- and post-operative resuscitation.

2-2-2 Surgical methods and means :

They are also very practical for children.

A. Operating protocol:

The child must be well covered, with only the abdomen exposed. A general anaesthetic, as is usual in paediatric abdominal surgery, will be administered. The operation must be carried out very gently. The aim is to remove the invaginated intestine. Resection should be reserved for the irreducible or complicated bowel (perforation, necrosis) and for treatment of the local cause (diverticulum, tumour, polyp).

1. Approach :

It is chosen according to the topography of the bulge, so palpation under general anaesthetic must be systematic, as it allows the invaginated bulge to be perceived.

Classically, laparotomy is performed via a transverse incision in the right iliac fossa, which can be enlarged to the midline if necessary. The bladder is often located in or near the right iliac fossa, whereas the median supraumbilical route is often recommended for other cases.

2. Treatment of lesions:

a. Manual reduction of intussusception:

It is best performed on an exteriorised bladder of the abdomen by applying gentle, constant pressure to the head of the bladder, without pulling on the upstream intestine, as this could rupture. Prior to exteriorisation of the bladder, warm serum should be prepared, and the intestines should be liberally infiltrated with xylocaine (non-adrenalised 1% xylocaine). After disinvagination, a few minutes are required to allow recovery of the ischemic intestinal segments. It is essential to ensure that there is no further intussusception and that no groove remains between the cecum and the ileum.

The graft is systematically checked, and the cause of intestinal intussusception must be sought and treated. Lastly, careful attention must be paid to reintegration.

b. Intestinal resection:

After disinvagination, if the sulcus remains ecchymotic, a new infiltration of the bowel is usually necessary; the intestinal segment rapidly returns to its normal colour and peristaltic waves are perceived, indicating its vitality. However, in the case of pre-perforative lesions or established necrosis, resection in a healthy area followed by immediate anastomosis is performed [59].

If reduction is not possible, resection is required, which will vary according to the type of invagination (ileo-ileal, ileo-colic or colo-colic), often with a terminal suture. Even if manual reduction of the sulcus is possible, this resection is performed as a matter of course to treat the local cause (Meckel's diverticulum).

3. The benefits of calioscopy:

Crelioscopy can be an alternative to conventional surgery and many authors report encouraging results. It should be noted that reduction of the bladder without pulling on the upstream bowel is not always easy and in half of cases results in surgical conversion [60].

4. Complementary treatments :

a. Appendectomy :

In principle, it is carried out. However, its necessity could be questioned in view of the morbidity induced by this procedure alone (fifth-day syndrome, occlusion on a flange). However, it remains a standard procedure, justified by, among other things, the inconvenience and source of error that such a scar could cause in a patient whose appendix has not been removed, or in order to limit the risk associated with the quality of its recovery. The need to fill in the child's health record correctly cannot be over-emphasised [61].

b. Ostomies :

In the case of peritonitis due to perforation of the bladder, immediate end-to-end anastomosis cannot be carried out due to the risk of the sutures coming loose, which is why stomas are indicated [58].

c. cmcopexy :

The various methods of attaching the c^cum to the parietal peritoneum or supporting the last loop of the ileum to the c^cum in order to prevent recurrence have not proved effective. Virtually all surgical teams have now abandoned them [34].

d. Parietal closure :

It must be done carefully to avoid evisceration or subsequent eventration. Drainage is not necessary except in cases of peritoneal effusion secondary to peritonitis.

e. Biopsy :

If there is a suspicion of digestive lymphoma, and if reduction of the sulcus is possible, surgery should avoid any attempt at tumour exeresis and be limited to diagnostic biopsies [62].

8- Indications:

- Barium enema: rarely indicated in children. In paediatrics, and in the majority of team-based services, the therapeutic sequence of a diagnostic enema followed by a therapeutic enema is the norm.

Patients must be monitored for recurrence. This can be done by opaque iterative enema and/or ultrasound. In these teams, surgery is only performed when the enema fails or is contraindicated.

- Surgery: This is indicated either in cases where barium enema is clearly contraindicated (peritoneal syndrome, explosive mel^na) or when enema is technically impossible.
- Reduction: This is indicated wherever possible.
- Resection: The indications for resection are less frequent in children than in adults, where it is more often necessary. These are :
- Sphacele evident before any manoeuvre on an invaginated segment (definite septicaemia),
- Irreversible ischemia after disinvagination;
- Failure of a complete disinvagination over the last few centimetres.
- Unsuccessful reversal of an invaginated diverticulum which still needs to be removed;
- Isolated benign or malignant tumour;
- Discovery of Peutz-Jeghers syndrome.

C- Post-operative monitoring :

This involves monitoring any operation involving bowel resection (at least of the appendix). Particular attention should be paid if there is a marked preoperative occlusive syndrome, or in the event of reintegration of a loop whose vitality was in doubt. The resumption of feeding is conditional on the clear resumption of transit [1].

Effective antibiotic prophylaxis against Gram-negative and anaerobic bacilli must be started as soon as the incision is made, and continued in the post-operative period until transit is resumed. Intestinal ischaemia and intraoperative manipulations encourage bacterial translocation, which can lead to septic shock in infants.

Post-operatively, recurrence after reduction surgery occurs in 1 to 4% of cases. It is therefore essential to warn parents of this risk of recurrence [63, 64].

D- Course and prognosis

The course and prognosis of the condition depend partly on the etiology of the intussusception, and partly on its complications (intestinal necrosis and perforation, septic shock). These complications are all the more important when there is a long delay in diagnosis.

Overall mortality from IIAS in African children is around 13%. This is most often due to delayed or missed diagnosis, but may also be due to the pathology responsible for secondary acute intussusception [65].

4 METHODOLOGY

111- METHODOLOGY:

3-1- Study framework:

The study was carried out in the paediatric surgery department of the Gabriel Toure University Hospital in Bamako (Mali).

3-1-1- Geographical location:

The CHU Gabriel Toure is located in the administrative centre of the city of Bamako (Commune III). It is bordered to the EAST by the popular Medinacoura district, to the WEST by the Ecole Nationale d'Ingenieurs (E.N.I), to the NORTH by the headquarters of the Army General Staff, and to the SOUTH by the Mali railway station. Formerly a dispensary, the CHU Gabriel Toure was set up as a hospital on 17 February 1959, bearing the name Gabriel Toure, in memory of a Sudanese medical student who died of plague contracted at his patient's bedside. The hospital became a university hospital when the University of Bamako opened in 1996.

The hospital's grounds include the surgical emergency department (SUC) in the south-west corner and the paediatric surgery department in the west of the Benitieni Fofana pavilion.

Description of the paediatric surgery department

3-1-2- Premises:

- The paediatric surgery department consists of:

S Eight (8) offices: one (1) for the head of department, four (4) for six (6) surgeons, one (1) for the major, one (1) for the interns and one (1) for the nurses and a secretariat.

S Seven (7) hospital wards (31 beds) including:

- Two (2) first-class rooms,
- Two (2) second-category rooms,
- Three (3) third-category rooms, including one reserved for brulees.

S The service is available:

- Seven (7) washbasins in the various offices;
- Two (2) containers for sharps: One (1) in the dressing room and the other (mobile) under the nurses' trolley.

The operating theatre is located on the first floor, in the EAST corner of the pavilion:

- Four (4) operating theatres, one of which is reserved for the paediatric surgery programme,
- One (1) changing room,
- One (1) reach box for patients to be operated on and

- One (1) post-interventional care room.
- Three (3) washbasins with two taps each for surgical hand washing

The emergency department: this comprises four sectors:

- First sector: reception and sorting;
- Second sector: two short-term hospitalisation units and eight cubicles;
- Third sector: an operating theatre which shares the different surgical specialities except gynaeco-obstetrics, a sterilisation room and a decontamination room;
- Fourth sector: a shredding room for conditioning before the operating theatre or before admission to the intensive care unit, and an on-call room.

3-1-3- Staff:

- There are six (6) paediatric surgeons, including two professors and one assistant professor.
- One (1) aesthetic and reconstructive surgeon.
- Two (2) medical assistants, one of whom is the major and the other the operating theatre assistant.
- Three (3) undergraduate nurses.
- Three (3) orderlies.
- Two (2) surface technicians.

Non-permanent staff:

Doctoral students acting as interns at the Faculty of Medicine and Dentistry (FMOS). The department also takes on post-graduate students, trainee doctors, external students from the Faculty of Medicine and Dentistry (FMOS), students from the National Institute for Training in Health Sciences (INFSS) and students from the Red Cross.

3-2- Activities:

3-2-1- The paediatric surgery department:

Outpatient consultations are held every day from Monday to Friday. Visits are made every morning, and inpatient admissions are made every day. Departmental staff meetings are held at 07:30, every day from Monday to Thursday. The general staff, which brings together all the surgical specialities, meets every Friday; the patients to be operated on are scheduled every Thursday. The various operations take place every Monday and Wednesday for the patients scheduled. The "Thesards" are divided between the different hospital wards, the operating theatre and the outpatients department.

3-2-2- Emergency department:

It is the first point of call for all surgical emergencies at Gabriel Toure University Hospital, with the exception of gynaecological and obstetric emergencies.

3-3- Patients:

They were recruited from the surgical emergency departments of the Gabriel Toure University Hospital.

3-3-1- Type and period of study:

This was a 6-year retrospective study from 1er January 2012 to 31 December 2017.

3-3-2- Study population:

All children aged 0-15 admitted to the paediatric surgery or emergency department.

3-3-3- Inclusion criteria:

Children with acute[1] secondary intestinal intussusception treated in our department.

3-3-4 Non-inclusion criteria:

- Children with acute intussusception[1] are managed in other departments.
- Idiopathic acute intestinal intussusception.
- Children whose medical records were incomplete.

3-4- Method:

All the patients recruited had benefited:

- An informed consent form for parents,
- A search for administrative data (surname, first name, age, address).
- A physical examination to look for significant signs (induced abdominal pain, localized tenderness, rectal bleeding, palpation of the bladder).
- Complementary examinations, in particular imaging (abdomino-pelvic ultrasound, PSA, CT scan)

Biology (Rhesus-grouping, haemoglobin level, etc.)

hematocrit, PT, APTT)

Anatomopathology (to analyse surgical specimens).

3-5- Support:

We have consulted:

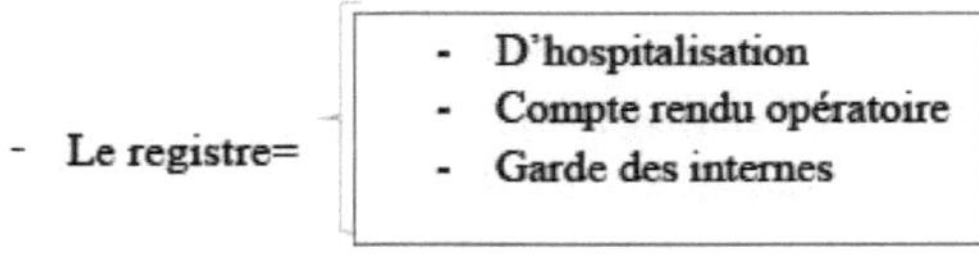

The register=

- Hospitalisation

- Surgical report

➢ Custody of interns

- The survey form: this contains variables distributed among the *S* Administrates data: age, gender, ethnicity, address, etc.

S Clinical and paraclinical parameters: functional signs, physical signs, additional tests;
S Operating sequences and
S Peroperative parameters.

3-6 Data entry and analysis :

The text and tables were entered using Microsoft Word.
The data were analysed using SPSS version 22 and epi-info version 7 software.
2. 1 The descriptive analysis consisted of calculating the absolute and relative frequencies for the qualitative variables, and the positioning and dispersion parameters for the quantitative variables using the 95% confidence interval.

3-7 Operational definitions :

- Consultation time: this corresponds to the time elapsed between the onset of signs and the date of admission to the wards where our study was carried out.
- Operating time: time elapsed between the date of admission and the date of surgery.
- Children: patients aged 0 to 15 are included in this category.
- Newborn: patient aged 0 to 28 days
- Infant: patient aged between 29 days and 30 months.
- Small children : Patients aged between 31 months and 78 months
- Older child: Patient aged between 79 months and 180 months.

5 RESULTS

RESULTS:

I. EPIDEMIOLOGICAL AND SOCIO-DEMOGRAPHIC DATA:

1. Frequency :

During the study period, 15572 patients were treated, including 225 cases of IIA and 35 cases of secondary origin, i.e. :

> 0.22% of consultations
> 0.82% of surgical activities (4267)
> 0.58% of hospital admissions (6001).
> 15.55% of intestinal invaginations.

2. Gender:

Table I: Breakdown of patients by sex

Gender	Workforce	Percentage
Male	**27**	**77,1**
Female	08	22,9
Total	**35**	**100**

Theex-ratio was3.4.

3. Age:

Table II: Age distribution of patients

Age	Workforce	Percentage
New-ne	01	02,9
Infant	12	34,3
Little child	**16**	**45,7**
Big kid	06	17,1
Total	**35**	**100**

The age group most affected was 2.6 years - 6.5 years, with 16 cases, or 45.7%. The mean age was 4.4±40.11 years, with extremes of 3 days and 14 years.

4. Provenance:

Table III: Breakdown of patients by origin

Origin	Workforce	Percentage
Bamako	**34**	**97,1**
Mopti	01	02,9
Total	**35**	**100**

One patient came to us from Mopti, representing 02.9% of cases.

5. Ethnicity:

Table IV: Distribution of patients by ethnic group

Ethnic group	Number	Percentage
Bambara	**1337 ,1**	
Peulh	0514 ,3	
Soninke	0514 ,3	
Malinke	0308,6	
Bobo	0205,7	
Senoufo	0205,7	
Other	0514 ,3	
Total	**35100**	

The Bambara ethnic group was the most represented in 37.1% of cases.

6. Reference:

Table V: Breakdown of patients by reference

Reference	Number	Percentage
Coming of their own accord	1028 ,6	
Doctor	**2571 ,4**	
Total	**35100**	

Over 28% of patients were not referred.

7. Reason for consultation:

Table VI: Breakdown of patients by reason for consultation

Reason for consultation	Number (n= 35)	Percentage
Abdominal pain2468	**.6**	
Vomiting2468 .6		
Rectorrhagia2057	.1	
Shutdown of materials and	gases0617	.1
Plaintive cries1748	,6	

In our study, abdominal pain and vomiting were the most common reasons for consultation, accounting for 68.6% of cases.

8. Evolutionary time:

Table VII: Breakdown of patients by admission time

Time to admission	Number	Percentage
1-3 days	**29**	**82,9**
4 - 6 days	09	17,1
Total	**35**	**100**

The average admission time was 2.7 ±1.29 days, with extremes of 1 day and 6 days.

9. General signs:

Table VIII: Distribution of patients according to general signs

General signs	Number of patients (n = 35)	Percentage
Conjunctivopalmoplantar heat18		**51,4**
Fievre08		22,9
Deshydrates04		11,4
Ictere01		02,9
Indetermines04		11,4

Conjunctivopalmoplantar pallor was found in 18 patients (51.4% of cases).

10. Functional signs :

Table IX: Distribution of patients according to functional signs

Functional signs	Number (n = 35)	Percentage
Abdominal pain24		**68,6**
Refusal to feed07		20
Crying and plaintive cries17		48,6
Vomiting24		**68,6**
Rectorrhagia20		57,1
Stop materials and gases06		17,1
Agitation04		11,4

In our study, abdominal pain and vomiting were the most common symptoms in 68.6% of cases.

11. Physical signs:

Table X: Distribution of patients according to physical signs

Physical signs	Number (n = 35)	Percentage
Reduced waterborne noise	2468 ,6	
Hydro-air noise abolished	1131 ,4	
Abdominal defence	1337 ,1	
Palpation of the bladder	**2160**	
Distended abdomen	1028 ,6	
Undistended abdomen	2571 ,4	
Vacuite de la FID	0205,7	

The invaginated bladder was palpable in 60% of cases.

12. Further tests:

12.1- Abdominal ultrasound:

Table XI: Distribution of patients according to abdominal ultrasound findings

Abdominal ultrasound	Workforce	Percentage
Image in cockade	06	17,1
Sandwich image	03	08,6
Undefined image	20	57,2
Ultrasound not performed	06	17,1

Total	35	100

Abdominal ultrasound was not performed in 17.1% of cases.

12.2- Unprepared abdominal X-ray (ASP):

Table XII: Distribution of patients according to PSA result

ASP	Workforce	Percentage
Image in grisaille	03	08,6
Image in air mould opacity	02	05,7
Image in poverty digestive aeration	01	02,8
ASP not implemented	**29**	**82,9**
Total	**35**	**100**

In 82.9% of cases, we did not request the ASP.

12.3- Grouping-Rhesus:

Table XIII: Distribution of patients according to Rhesus grouping result

Groupage-Rhesus	Workforce	Percentage
A +	**16**	**45,7**
AB +	01	2,9
B -	01	2,9
B +	09	25,7
O +	08	22,8
Total	**35**	**100**

Most of our patients were group **"A"** and rhesus **"+"** with a percentage of 45.7% of cases.

13. Diagnosis:

13. 1- Preoperative diagnosis:

Table XIV: Distribution of patients by preoperative diagnosis

Preoperative diagnosis	Number of patients	Percentage
Occlusion on flange	02	05,7
Acute intestinal invagination	**30**	**85,6**
Atresie du grele	01	02,9
Acute intestinal obstruction	01	02,9
Appendicular peritonitis	01	02,9
Total	**35**	**100**

The diagnosis of acute intestinal intussusception was made in 85.6% of cases.

13.1- Intraoperative diagnosis:

Table XV: Breakdown of patients by peroperative diagnosis

Intraoperative diagnosis patients	**Number**	**ofPercentage**
I. Ileo-ileale10		**28,5**
I. Colo-colic08		22,9
I. Ileo-colique03		8,5
I. Caeco-colique01		2,9
I. Ileo-caeco-colique08		22,9
I. Ileo-caecale05		14,3
Total35		**100**

In our study, the "Ileo-ileal" form was the most prevalent in 28.5% of cases.

<u>NB:</u> I = Invagination

14. Approach:

Table XVI: Breakdown of patients by approach route

Approach	Workforce	Percentage
Median above and below the umbilicus	05	14,3
Transverse para-umbilical	**30**	**85,7**
Total	**35**	**100**

The transverse para-umbilical route was used in 85.7% of cases.

15. Operating technique:

Table XVII: Distribution of patients according to surgical technique

Operating technique	Workforce	Percentage
Manual disinvagination1028	.6	
Resection anastomosis2365	**,7**	
Stomy0205	,7	
Total35100		

Anastomotic resection was the operative technique used in 65.7% of cases.

16. Etiology:

Table XVIII: Breakdown of patients by etiology

Etiology	Workforce	Percentage
Meckel's diverticulum	**10**	**28,5**
Intestinal polyps	**10**	**28,5**
Malignant lymphoma	01	2,9
Gluten intolerance	08	22,9
Cystic fibrosis	01	2,9
Post-operative IIA	02	5,7
Chemotherapy	01	2,9

Thermal burn	02	5,7
Total	**35**	**100**

Meckel's diverticulum and intestinal polyps were the main causes of secondary acute intussusception in 28.5% of our patients.

17. Length of hospital stay:

Table XIX: Breakdown of patients by length of hospital stay (in days)

Length of stay	Number of patients	Percentage
04 to 0720		**57,1**
08 to 1410		28,6
15 to 2001		02,9
> 2104		11,4
Total35		**100**

The average length of hospital stay for our patients was 9.24±5.36 days, with extremes of 4 days and 25 days.

18. Follow-up operations :

18.1- Immediate surgical follow-up

Table XX: Distribution of patients according to immediate post-operative effects

Follow-up operations immediate	Workforce	Percentage
Suppuration04		**11,4**
Eventration02		05,7
Evisceration01		02,9
Occlusion01		02,9
Simple suites27		77,1
Total35		**100**

Parietal suppuration was the main complication at the surgical site in 11.4% of our patients.

18.2- Late surgical follow-up :

Table XXI: Distribution of patients according to late post-operative effects

Late surgical follow-up	Workforce	Percentage
Decedes	03	08,6
Living	**32**	**91,4**
Total	**35**	**100**

The post-operative course was straightforward in 91.4% of cases.

6 COMMENTS AND DISCUSSION

COMMENTS AND DISCUSSION

1-Methodology :

This was a retrospective study of secondary acute intestinal intussusception in children, from 1er January 2012 to 31 December 2017, i.e. a period of 6 years in the paediatric surgery department of the CHU Gabriel Toure.

We have encountered a number of difficulties, including

> Lack of sufficient information in certain files

> Retention of files

> The non-availability of certain emergency tests (ultrasound, CT scan, CBC, blood ionogram, PT and aPTT)

> Frequent stock-outs of kit and the low purchasing power of some patients.

2-Epidemiology :

2-1 Frequency:

Over a period of 6 years, our study involved 225 patients, 35 of whom presented with secondary intestinal intussusception in children, representing a frequency of 15.55% of all intestinal intussusceptions operated on in the paediatric surgery department of the Gabriel Toure University Hospital. This frequency is within the range of 2.5% to 18% reported in the literature [4].

2-2. Breakdown by gender:

Table XXII: Breakdown by sex ratio and authors

Authors	Duration study	Number of cases	Male	Female	Ratio
NOUIRA [27], Tunis 2010	15 years old	25 cases	18	07	02,57
BENGARAI [28], Rabat 2013	43 months	21 cases	14	07	02,00
MHANNA [9], Fes 2015	48 months	13 cases	10	03	3,33
ENEHWI [8], Marrakech 2016	05 years old	13 cases	08	05	1,60
Our 2017 study	06 years old	35 cases	27	08	3,4

Acute intestinal intussusception is most often described in gargons.

This male predominance could be explained by the greater lymphoid tissue in the gargon than in the girl.

We recorded a sex ratio of 3.4. This rate is comparable to that of other authors NOUIRA, BENGARAI, MHANNA and ENEHWI [27], [28], [9] and [8].

4- Age distribution:

In our study, we recorded only one case of neonatal secondary IIA.

Table XXIII: Distribution of patients according to age and authors

Authors	Average age	Patients aged over two years
WAJEEH UDDIN [47], Karachi 2010	2.15 years	Less than 50
W. BENGARAI [28], Rabat 2013	6.5 years	72 %
MHANNA [9], Fes 2015	4 years	69 %
ENEHWI [8], Marrakech 2016	2.10 years	69 %
Our 2017 study	4.4 years	62,8 %

The average age of our patients was 4.4 years. This is the age of the child. WAJEE UDDIN [47] and ENEHWI [9] recorded infants instead. This difference could be explained by the occurrence of secondary acute intestinal intussusception in children over 2 years of age and exceptionally in infants under 2 months of age.

II. CLINICAL STUDY:

Table XXV: Symptomatic triad in secondary II

Authors	Symptomatic triad	P
WAJEEH UDDIN [47], Karachi 2010	15/19 (78,9 %)	0,2195
W. BENGARAI [28], Rabat 2013	7/21(33,3 %)	0,1821
MHANNA [9], Fes 2015	3/13(23 %)	0,2549
ENEHWI [8], Marrakech 2016	1/13(07 %)	0,3826
Our 2017 study	22/35(62,8 %)	-

In our study, the classic symptomatic triad of II (paroxysmal painful attacks, vomiting and rectal discharge) was noted in 62.8% of cases. This rate is comparable to that of other studies [28, 47, 9, 8], (p = 0.1384).

In secondary acute intestinal intussusception, the classic picture is not always found.

Table XXVI: Signs of physical examination during secondary II

Authors	AEG	Abdominal mass	Rectorrhagia	Shutdown of materials and gases	Abdominal distension
BENGARAI [28], Rabat 2013	52,4 % P = 0,1722	43 % P = 0,1737	23,8 % P = 0,2007	No data	No data
MHANNA [9], Fes 2015	23 % P = 0,2549	7,5 % P = 0,3825	15 % P = 0,2936	No data	No data
ENEHWI [8], Marrakech 2016	35,8 % P = 0,2175	25,3 % P = 0,2505	54,54 % P = 0,2174	18,7 % P = 0,2797	28,7 % P = 0,2295
Our study 2017	22,8 %	60 %	57,1 %	17,1 %	28,6 %

In acute secondary intestinal intussusception, vomiting and refusal to nurse very rapidly lead to alteration of the patient's general condition (AEG), which we noted in 22.8% of cases. This rate is comparable to that of other authors: BENGARAI [28], MHANNA [9] and ENEHWI [8].
Palpation of the intussusception bladder is not always evident on physical examination because of abdominal distension, and we only have it in 60% of our patients. This rate is also comparable to that of other authors: BENGARAI [28], MHANNA [9] and ENEHWI [8].
Jaundice is only evident when intestinal distress sets in, and we recorded it in 57.1% of cases. This can be explained by the delay in diagnosis. This rate is comparable to that of other authors: BENGARAI [28], MHANNA [9] and ENEHWI [8].
We noted 17.1% of cessation of fluid and gas and 28.6% of abdominal distension. This rate is comparable to that of ENEHWI [8] except that BENGARAI [28] and MHANNA [9] did not conduct studies on this subject.
The clinical symptoms are varied and often misleading: acute occlusive symptoms, sub-occlusive symptoms with a progressive onset lasting from a few days to a few weeks; non-specific abdominal syndromes (cessation of transit, diffuse abdominal pain, vomiting, digestive bleeding), sometimes evolving over several months, with or without changes in general condition [37,38].

II. ADDITIONAL EXAMINATIONS

1. Unprepared X-ray of the abdomen:

The first radiologically diagnosed intussusception was described by Lehmann in 1914, and since then unprepared abdominal X-rays have been widely used to help diagnose II, especially in children [1].

Table XXVII: Breakdown by ESL score

Authors	NHA	Vacuite of the IDF	Rare digestive tract infections	Opacity of the pudding	P
MHANNA [9], Fes 2015	38,4 %	23 %	15,38 %	07,5 %	0,2227
ENEHWI [8], Marrakech 2016	33,8 %	05,95 %	No data	10,44 %	0,2278
Our study	17,1 %	08,6 %	02,8 %	05,7 %	-

Despite its usefulness, standard radiography lacks sensitivity and many false negatives are encountered, even in the absence of radiographic signs of intussusception.

In our study, an unprepared abdominal X-ray (UPX) was performed in 06 of our patients. It contributed to the diagnosis by revealing hydro-aeric levels characterising the occlusion site in 17.1% of cases. This rate is comparable to that of other authors, MHANNA [9] and ENEHWI [8].

2. Abdominal ultrasound :

Bowerman was the first to describe the ultrasound appearance of invaginations in the 1980s. It is a rapid, non-invasive examination that is easy to perform and reproducible, and represents the key to diagnosis, with some authors now giving it a sensitivity of close to 100% [32, 33]. The only limitations of ultrasound investigation are the gaseous interposition that may be encountered in the major occlusive syndromes of advanced or ileo-iliac IIA.

Table XXVIII: Contribution of ultrasound in secondary IIA

Authors	Number of ultrasounds	Number of IIA confirmesa ultrasound	Percentage	P
MHANNA[9], Fes 2015	12	10	92,3 %	0,2549
ENEHWI [8], Marrakech 2016	10	07	76,9 %	0,2176
Our 2017 study	29	09	82,9 %	-

In our study, abdominal ultrasound was performed in 29 patients, i.e. 82.9% of cases, and confirmed the diagnosis of II in 09 patients, i.e. 25.71% of cases. This rate does not differ from that of other authors MHANNA [9] and ENEHWI [8].

IV. TYPE OF INVAGINATION Type of intussusception

Table XXIX: Type of intussusception according to authors

Authors	Ileo-ileale	Colonic	Ileo- caeco-colic	Ileo-caecale	Ileo-colic Transvalvular
MHANNA [9], Fes 2015	8/13(61,53 %) P =0,2205	1/13(07,7 %) P =0,3826	1/13(07,7 %) P =0,3826	-	3/13(23,07 %) P =0,2545
Our study 2017	10/35(28,5 %)	8/35(22,9 %)	8/35(22,9 %)	5/35(14 ,3 %)	3/35(08,5 %)

In secondary intestinal invaginations, the most frequently found forms are : Ileo-ileal and colo-colic.

In our series, the most predominant form was 'Ileo-ileale', which was also the most highly rated in all the series.

V. Etiologies

Table XXX: Etiological factors according to authors

Authors	Diverticulum de Meckel	Digestive polyps	Malignant lymphoma	cwliaquc disease	Post-op	Cystic fibrosis
MHANNA [9], Fes 2015	5/13(38 %) P :0,2224	-	2/13(15 %) P :0,2937	1/13(07 %) P :0,3826	-	
ENEHWI [8], Marrakech 2016	5/13(38 %) P :0,2224	1/13(08 %) P :0,3826	4/13(31 %) P :0,2340	-		
Ourstudy 2017	10/35(28,5 %)	10/35(28, 5%)	1/35(02,9%)	8/35(22,9%)	2/35(05,7 %)	1/35(02,9%)

Meckel's diverticulum was the main cause in all series [9] and [8].

This could be explained by the sampling, as statistically it does not differ from that found by other authors MHANNA [9] and ENEHWI [8].

We also recorded other cases: one (1) case of chemotherapy and two (2) cases during hospitalisation for thermal burns by hot water and flame.

NB: In our cases, the resections were sent for anatomopathological examination, sweat tests and biopsies, which confirmed the causes suspected peroperatively or beforehand.

VI. Treatment

Table XXXI: Treatment according to authors

Authors	Manual	Resection	Stoma

	disinvagination	anastomosis	
W. BENGARAI [28], Rabat 2013	5/21(23,8 %) P :0,2007	16/21(76,2 %) P :0,2007	00 %
MHANNA [9], Fes 2015	00 %	13/13(100 %) P :1	00 %
ENEHWI [8], Marrakech 2016	8/13(59,5 %) P :0,2205	5/13(37,71 %) P :0,2224	1/13(07,6 %) P :0,3826
Our 2017 study	10/35(28,6 %)	23/35(65,7 %)	2/35(05,7 %)

In our study, anastomotic resection was performed in 23 of our patients, i.e. 65.7% of cases, a rate comparable to that of other authors BENGARAI, MHANNA and ENEHWI [28, 9, 8].

This result could be explained by :

- The etiology of IIAS in particular.

VII. EVOLUTION:

The morbidity of this condition is linked to the complications of intussusception (necrosis, perforation and septic shock). These complications are all the more significant when there is a long delay in diagnosis, but they also depend on the etiology of the intussusception. Morbidity is also linked to surgical complications (complications of anaesthesia, wall abscesses, risk of occlusion on a flange).

In our study, we identified four (4) cases of parietal suppuration, two (2) cases of postoperative eventration, one (1) case of postoperative evisceration and one (1) case of flange occlusion which were managed early with satisfactory outcome.

Overall mortality from IIAS in children in Africa is around 13% [65].

In our study, we recorded three (3) deaths among our patients, one due to cystic fibrosis and the other two due to thermal burns caused by hot water (estimated at 39%) and flame (estimated at 52%), i.e. a mortality rate of 8.6%, whereas that of MHANNA T [9] was favourable in 100% of cases, i.e. a mortality rate of 0%, and that of ENEHWI. AMED [8] was also unfavourable in 15.4% of cases, i.e. 2 deaths including one case of septic shock and the other case of septic shock on lymphoma.

7 CONCLUSION AND RECOMMENDATIONS

CONCLUSION :

Acute intestinal intussusception[1] is a relatively frequent abdominal emergency in our context. It is difficult to diagnose in the absence of specific additional investigations. It is diagnosed mainly peroperatively. Digestive tumours were the most frequent etiology in our study. Early management of the patient will improve his vital prognosis. Treatment is surgical and, above all, adapted to the etiology. It is also often multidisciplinary.

RECOMMENDATIONS :

We would like to make a few recommendations:

> To the authorities :

- Making access to healthcare more equitable between regions and between social categories.
- Train enough specialists in child surgery, paediatrics, paediatric intensive care and radiology.
- Equipping hospitals with appropriate diagnostic and therapeutic resources.

> For healthcare professionals:

- Carefully examine any child presenting with tiiguc abdominal pain .[1]
- Refer patients as quickly as possible to referral facilities.
- Strengthening interdisciplinary collaboration involving paediatric surgeons, paediatricians, intensive care units and radiologists.

> To the public :

- Any intermittent abdominal pain in children should be treated promptly.
- Avoid self-medication.

Bibliography:

1-Franchi.S ;Martelli.H ;Paye-jaouen.A ;Goldzmidt.D ; Pariente. D.
Acute intestinal intussusception in infants and children.
EMC-pediatrie 2 (2005) 45-57.

2- Sarnacki .S ; Sayegh.N ; Martelli.H.
IIA in infants and children. EMC pediatrie; 4-018-P-10, 1996,6P.

3- MEZANE SAIDA et al. Acute intestinal invagination in infants and children [These Med]. Fes : Universite Sidi Mohamed Ben Abdellah; 2011. P 162.

4- Aubrespy P, Derlon S, Alessandrini P, et al.
Acute intestinal invagination[1] in infants and children. Analysis of 125 surgically treated cases. ChirPediatr 1983;24:392-5.

5-HuppertzHI ; Soriano-Gabarro M ; Grimprel E ; et al.
Intussusception among young children in Europe.Pediatr Infect Dis J 2006; 25 (Suppel 1) S 22 - 9.

6- Sami A. Unusual cause of intussusception: diffuse large B-cell non Hodgkin's lymphoma: a case report and review. *Eur Med Pharmacol SCI* 2012 Dec; 16(14):1938-46.

7-Ongom PA, Opio CK, Kijjambu SC.
An etiology and treatment of children intussusception in a tertiary Sub-Saharan Hospital: a 10-year retrospective study. BMC Gastroenterol. 2014 May; 14(1):86.

8- ENEHWI AHMEDOU. Secondary acute intestinal intussusception in children. [These Med]. Marrakech : CADI-AYYAD University ; 2016. P 166. N° = 95.

9- T. MHANNA. Secondary acute intestinal intussusception in children: 13 cases. [These Med]. Fes : Universite Sidi Mohamed Ben Abdellah ; 2015. P 166. N° = 019.

10- TRAORE D, SISSOKO F, ONGOIBA N, TRAORE I, TRAORE AK, KOUMARE AK.
Intussusception: diagnosis, morbidity and mortality in a developing country. Journal of visceral surgery June 2012; 149(3): 211-4.

11- BOUALI O, ABBO O, IZARD P, BAUNIN P, GALINIER P. Acute intestinal invagination[1] in infants and children.
EMC - Urgence. 2012 September ; Volume 16, Issue 3 - Pages 1 - 9.

12- Barbette P. (.Envies chirurgies et anatomiques. Geneva: Francois Miege; 1674 522p.

13- Hutchinson J. A. Successful case of abdominal section for intussusception.

Proc R Med ChirSoc 1873;7:195.

14- Ravitch MM. Intussusception. In: Ravitch MM, Welch KJ, Benson C, Aberdeen E, Randolph JG, editors. Pediatric surgery. Chicago: Year1986 Book Medical Publisher p. 868-82.

15- Gross RE.
The surgery of infancy and Child Hood.
Philadelphia: WB Saunders; 1953 297p.

16- Ein SH, Stephens CA.
Intussusception: 354 cases in 10 years.
J PediatrSurg 1971; 6:16-27

17- R. AMRANI, S. MESSAOUDI, A. SEDDIKI, N. TAZI.
Acute intestinal invagination[1] revealing celiac disease in a 7-month-old infant. Journal of pediatrics and puericulture (2015) 28, 80 - 82.

18- PISACANE A; CARACCIOLO G; DELUCA U; GRILLO G et Coll.
Infant feeding and intussusception. 1993;
Vol 123; N°4, pages 593-595.

19- Ong NT, Beasley SW.
The lead point in intussusception. J PediatrSurg 1990;25:640-3.

20- WEST .K. W; STEPHENS .B; RESORLA .F .J; et al.
Post operative Intussusception: Experience With 36 Cases in Children ; Surgery (October) 1988;Vol 104, pages 781-787.

21- DE VRIES S, SLEEBOOM C, ARONSON D.C.
Postoperative intussusception in children.
British Journal of Surgery.1999; 86:81-3.

22- YU ZUO BAI, HUI CHEN, WEI LIN.
A special type of postoperative intussusception: ileo-ileal intussusception after surgical reduction of ileocolic intussusception in infants and children. Journal of Pediatric Surgery.2009; 44- 755-58.

23- NIAUDET. P ; BENAMAYO. J. P.
Systemic diseases with renal involvement;
Archives de pediatrie ; 2006 ; N° 13 ; pages 596-603.

24- OUEDRAOGO YEWAGNA DIT MAHAMADI.
Acute intestinal intussusception: epidemiological, clinical and therapeutic aspects. [These Med]. Burkina-Faso: Universitaire Yalgado OUEDRAOGO et Charles DE GAULLE de Ouagadougou; 2012. P 120. N° = 145.

25- Patte C, Philip T, Rodary C, et al.
High survival rate in advanced stage B-cell lymphomas and leukemias without CNS involvement with a short intensive. Results of a polychemotherapyrandomised trial from the French Pediatric Oncology Society

(SFOP). J Clin
Oncol 1991;9: 123-32.
26- Abou-Nukta F, Gutweiler J, Khaw J, Yavorek G.
Giant lipoma causing a colo-colonic intussusception.
Am Surg. 2007;73(4):417.
27- NOUIRA F, YENGUI H, BEN AHMED Y, CHARIEG A, KHEMAKHEM R, GHORBEL S.
Secondary intestinal intussusception: 25 paediatric cases.
Archive de pediatrie. 2010 June; Volume 17, Issue 6, Supplement 1-109.
28- WIFAK BENGARAI. Les invaginations secondaires chez L'enfant a propos de 21 cas aux urgences chirurgicales pediatriques. [TheseMed], Rabat: Universite Mohamed V-Souissi; 2013. P 180. N° = 98.
29- P. PETIT, J.P. PRACROS.
The role of ultrasound in digestive emergencies in children. J Radiol 2001; 82:764-78.
30- BINES J.E., IVANOFF B., JUSTICE F., MULHOLLAND K.
Clinical case definition for the diagnosis of acute intussusceptions.
J PediatrGastroenterolNutr 2004; 39:511-8.
31- RAMACHANDRAN P., VINCENT P., PRABHU S., SRIDHARAN S.
Rectal prolapse of intussusception, a single institution's experience.
Eur J PediatrSurg, 2006; 16:420-2.
32- Pracros JP, Tran-Minh VA, Morin DE.
Acute intestinal intussusception in children: contribution of ultrasonography.
Ann Radiol 1987; 30:525-30.
33- Hasegawa T, Sumimura J, Mizutani S, TazukeY, Okuda S, Dezawa T.
The doughnut sign: an ultrasound finding in pediatric intestinal Burkitt's lymphoma. PediatrSurgInt 1998;13:297-8.
34- Leon K Eisen, John D Cunningham, Arthur H Aufses Jr.
Intussusception in children: Institutional Review.
J Am CollSurg 1999;188:390-395.
35-Lebeau R, Koffi E, Diane B, Amani A, Kouassi JC.
Acute intestinal invaginations in children: analysis of a series of 20 cases. Ann Chir2006; 131: 447-50.
36- FATIH EROL .M; SEVKI KARAKAYALI .A; OZER .S; YILDIZ .M
Mucosa-associated lymphoid tissue lymphoma of the ileum as the cause of an intestinal invagination.Journal of Pediatric Surgery. 2008; N° 43, pages: 13-15.
37- Ein SH, Stephens CA, Shandling B, Filler RM.
Due to lymphoma. J PediatrSurg 1986;21:786-8.

38-Brichon P, BertrandY, Plantaz D.
Burkitt's lymphoma revealed by acute intestinal invagination[1] in children. Ann Chir 2001;126:649- 53.
39- Pui CH, Evans WE.
Treatment of childhood acute lymphoblastic leukemia.
N Engl J Med 2006;354:166-78.
40- Redaelli A, Laskin BL, et al.
A systematic literature review of the clinical and epidemiological burden of acute lymphoblastic leukaemia (ALL).Eur J Cancer Care (Engl) 2005;14:53-62. M. Schiffa, H. Ogier de Baulnya. Macrocytosis of metabolic origin.
Archives of Pediatrics 2013;20:180-182.
41- Valayer. J.
Congenital malformations of the duodenum and intestine ;
EMC- pediatrie, 4-017-B-10,2006.
42-NOURI A, BELGHITH M, MEKKI M, BEN ATTIA M, HOUISSA T.
Digestive duplications in children. About 24 cases.
RevMaghrebPediatr. 1993; 3-17-21.
43- Mazzola a, D. Balas b, C. Deminiere c, N. Grenier d, H. De Clermont e, F. Comby f, J.-M. Ferriere a, G. Pasticier a et Al.
Heterotopic gastric and vesical siege: a clinical case at the crossroads of embryology and histopathology. Doi : 10. 1016 / j. Purol. 2010. 05. 004. N° 4, Pages 296-299.
44- Fahd. Ouchen.
Acute intestinal intussusception in infants and children at the TETOUAN provincial hospital, (2007). Les invaginations intestinales secondaires chez les enfants [These Med]. Fes : Universite Sidi Mohamed Ben Abdellah. 2015. P 150. N° = 019.
45- ZANELLI .S; DI MAIO .M; DODAT .H et Coll ;
Acute intestinal invagination[1] .
Archives de Pediatrie, September 1995; Volume 2, Issue 9; pages 897-898.
46- BEN MERIEM .C; HAMMAMI .S; CHOUCHANE .S etColl ;
Rheumatoid purpura in children: 67 cases ;
Journal de pediatrie et de puericulture ; 2006; N° 19, pages 323-327
47- Wajeeh.UDDIN; MANDLAL.K; JAVED.A; TALAT.M; NOSHAD. A
An audit of non-idiopathic intussusception in children.
Jlumis. 2010 September - December; Vol 09 N°= 03-134-36.
48- Mohamed HAMID. Management of acute intestinal intussusception in infants and children. [These Med]. Marrakech : CADI- AYYAD University ; 2011. P 123. N° = 77.

49- Galinier. P, Izard .P, Juricie .M, Kern .D, Domenech .B, Baunin .C, Puget.
C, Vaysse .P. Acute intestinal invagination in infants and children;
EMC, urgency, 24-300-C-10, 2007.
50-EKLOF O; HARTELIUS H.
Reliability of the abdominal plain film diagnosis in pediatric patient with
Suspected intussusception Pediatr. Radiol. 1980; vol. 9; pages 199-206.
51- Kull E, Blanchet E, Beau P.
Intestinal invagination and coeliac disease: a case report.
GastroenterolClinBiol 2003; 27: 1043-5.
52- Essomba .A, Mefire .A.C, Fokou .M, Ouassouo .P.M, Esiene. A ,Abolo .L.M, Malong .E.E ; Les abdomen aigus d'etiologie parasitaire: analyse d'une serie retrospective de 135 cas . Annales de chirurgie 131 (2006) ,194-197.
53- E. DUTOIT.
Trichocephales and Trichcephalosis.
EMC - Pediatrics 2 (2005) 355-362.
54-ARCHANE **M.I, SEBTI M, ALAOUI T, BALAFREJ A, TOLOUNE F, AHAYON V.**
Digestive disorders in progressive pulmonary tuberculosis.
In 46e Congres Frangais de Medecine, Marrakech, Masson, 1987: 23-36.
55- LAMDAOUAR BOUAZZAOUI N.
"Infectious diseases of newborns, infants and children.
Rabat, Editions Nouvelles, 1989: 399-428.
56-M. Kisra, I. Azzouzi; F. Ettaybi; M. Benhamou.
Intestinal invagination caused by a Trichobezoard.
Medecine du Maghreb 2001, N° 86.
57-E. Youssef. Acute intestinal invagination secondary to trichobezoard in children. Pan Afr Med J. 2014; 17: 31.
58- EL KAOUI .H; BOUCHENTOUF .SM; SALL.I; SAIR. K et Coll.
Intestinal invagination on fibro-inflammatory polyp of Vanek ;
Clinical and Biological Gastroenterology; November 2007, Vol 31, Issue 11, pages 978-979.
59- M. BEN AMEUR et al.
Secondary intestinal intussusception in children: 14 cases [These Med]. [These Med].Rabat :Universite Mohamed V - Souissi ; 2008.P 110. N° = 173.
60- SCHIER F. Experience with laparoscopy in the treatment of intussusception. Journal of Pediatric Surgery 1997; 32: 1713-4.
61- KHEN-DUNLOP N., SARNACKI S., SAYEGH-DAGHER N.
Acute intestinal invagination[1] in infants and children.

EMC, Gastro-enterology, 9-044-I-10, 2008.

62- K. MAAZOUN, M. MEKKI, L. SAHNOUN, S. HAFSA, M. BEN BRAHIM, M. BELGHITH, A. ZAKHAMA, R. JOUINI, M. GOLLI, I. KRICHENE, A. NOURI.
Unusual causes of acute intestinal intussusception[1] : about 27 cases ;
Archives de pediatrie 14 (2007) 4-9.

63- HUPPERTZ .H.I; SORIANO-GABARRO .M; GRIMPREL .E; FRANCO .E et Coll.
Intussusception Among Young Children in Europe The Pediatric Infectious Disease Journal. January 2006; Volume 25, pages 22-29

64-V. Juliana, M. Biardb, A. Labbe, F. Amata.
Acute intestinal intussusception[1] atypical Archives de Pediatrie 2012; 19 : 526 - 527.

65- Steele AD, Patel M, Cunliffe NA, Bresee JS, Borgstein E, Parashar UD. Workshop on intussusception in African countries -- meeting report.Vaccine. 2012 Apr 27;30Suppl 1:A185 - 9. doi: 10.1016/j.vaccine.2011.10.004.

66-K. Bentama; I. Chemalal; M. Benabbou et al. Acute intestinal invagination consecutive to a graft lipoma: a case report and review of the literature. Pan Africanmedical journal. 2012; 12: 98.

67- PR OLIVIER REINBERG.
Abdominal pain in children: when should you call the surgeon?
Rev Med Suisse 2012; 8: 2092 - 7.

APPENDICES

Conclusion:

Acute intestinal intussusception[1] is a relatively frequent abdominal emergency in our context. It is difficult to diagnose in the absence of specific additional investigations. It is diagnosed mainly peroperatively. Digestive tumours were the most frequent etiology in our study. Early management of the patient will improve his vital prognosis. Treatment is surgical and, above all, adapted to the etiology. It is also often multidisciplinary.

Key words : II, IIAS, DM, paediatric surgery, Mali.

Survey form

Observation sheet n°: /_

Medical file n° /,

I. Socio-demographic data:

1. ***Name:***
2. ***First name***
3. ***Age: 1- Newborn // 2- Infant //3- 3 to 9 years old //4-10 to 15 years old //***
4. ***Sex: 1- Male /___/ 2- Female /___/ /***
5. ***Ethnic group: 1- Bambara /__ / 2- Malinke /__ / 3- Peulh /__ / 4- Bobo /__ / 5- Minyanka // 6- Senoufo // 7- Soninke / / 8- Dogon / / 9- Sonrhai /__ /10- Maure //11- Kakolo //12- Other to specify:***
6. ***Nationality: 1- Malian /__ / 2- Non-Malian /_ /***
7. ***Contact (Address):***
8. ***Origin: 1- Kayes /__ / 2- Koulikoro /__ / 3- Sikasso /__ / 4- Segou /__ / 5- Mopti /__ / 6- Tombouctou /__ / 7- Gao /__ / 8- Kidal /__ / 9- Bamako /__ / 10- Other:***
9. ***Address by: 1- Doctor /__ / 2- Nurse /__ / 3- Parent(s) /__ / 4- In hospital / /5- Other to specify:***
10. ***The date of admission:***
11. ***The release date:***

II. Antecedents:

1- Staff:

a- Medical:

1- Digestive tumour:
2- Purpura rheumato'ide:
3- Hemolytic uremic syndrome:
4- Cystic fibrosis:
5- Hemangioma:
6- Abdominal trauma:
7- Thermal burns
8- Chemotherapy:
9- Calia disease:
10- Other causes to be specified:

*b- **Surgical:***

11- Meckel's diverticulum

12- Digestive duplication

13- Intestinal polyp

14- Opere (es): 1- Yes /__ / 2- No /___ / 3- If yes, for which pathology / .

15- Others to be specified:

*c- **Family:***

16- Father:

17- Mere:

18- Co11aTёгaux:

19- Others to specify:

III. Reason for consultation:

a- Abdominal pain: 1- Yes / / 2- No / /

b- Crying and screaming: 1- Yes / / 2- No / /

c- Vomiting: 1- Yes / / 2- No / /

d- Refusal to feed: 1- Yes // 2- No //

e- Rectorrhagia: 1- Yes / / 2- No ∠ /

f- Shut-off of materials and gases: 1- Yes // 2- No //

g- Agitation: 1- Yes / / 2- No / /

h- Others to specify:

2- Signs ∂ёпёmux:

a- Condition ∂ёпёm1:1- Good / / 2- Fair / / 3- Poor / /

b- Fever (TвmpёM^в зuрё^u^ a 38° c): 1- Yes // 2- No //

c- Dёshydration: 1- Yes // 2- No //

d- Heat: 1- Yes // 2- No //

e- State of shock: 1- Yes / / 2- No / /

f- Others to specify:

3- Functional signs:

a- Dёlais of consultation:

b- Pain: 1- Yes / / 2- No ∠ /

c- Plaintive cries: 1- Yes / / 2- No / /

d- Vomiting: 1- Yes / /2- No ∠ /

e- Rectorrhagia: 1- Yes / / 2- No ∠ /

f- Others to specify:

4- Physical signs:

a- Inspection:

1- Abdominal distension: a- Yes / / b- No ∠ /

2- Bloated abdomenё: a- Yes // b- No //

3- Abdominal tuck: a- Yes ∠ / b- No / /

4- Ecchymosis: a- Yes ∠ / b- No / /

5- Pёtёchies: a- Yes // b- No //

6- Others to specify:

b- Palpation:

1- *Pain provoked: a- Yes / / b- No /_ /*

2- *Abdominal mass: a- Yes / / b- No / /*

3- *Vacuite de la FID: a- Yes // b- No //*

4- *Others to be specified:*

c- Percussion:

1- *Tympany: a- Yes ∠ / b- No //*

2- *Sub-matite: a- Yes ∠ / b- No ∠ /*

3- *Matter: a- Yes ∠ / b- No ∠ /*

d- Auscultation: Hydro-air noises,

1- *Present /___ / 2- Diminished / / 3- Abolished / /*

e- Rectal examination:

1- *Rectorrhagia: a- Yes / / b- No //*

2- *Invagination pudding: a- Yes / / b- No ∠ /*

3- *Prolapse of the bladder: a- Yes ∠ / b- No / /*

4- *Empty rectum: a- Yes / / b- No / /*

5- *Others to be specified:*

IV. Paraclinical tests:

1- Biological tests:

- *Grouping: ; Rhesus:*
- *CBC: 1- Normal / / 2- Abnormal //*
- *Anemia: 1- Yes / / 2- No / /*
- *Hyperleukocytosis: 1- Yes / / 2- No ∠ /*
- *CRP: 1- Normal / / 2- Abnormal / /*
- *VS: 1- Normal / / 2- Abnormal / /*
- *PT: 1- Normal /___ / 2- Abnormal /___ /*
- *APTT: 1- Normal ∠ / 2- Abnormal / /*
- *Blood ionogram: 1- Normal /___ / 2- Abnormal / /*
- *Uree: 1- Normale /___ / 2- Diminuee ∠ / 3- High / /*
- *Creatininemia: 1- Normal /___ / 2- Decreased /___ / 3- High / /*
- *Clearance: 1- Normal /___ / 2- Decreased /___ / 3- High /___ /*
- *Other to be specified:*

2- Radiological signs:

- ***Ultrasound:***
  - *Cross-section of the invagination flange: Cocarde image /__ /*
  - *Longitudinal section of the invagination flange: Sandwich image /__ /*
- ***ASP:***
  - *Image in "Grisaille de la FID": ∠ /*
  - *Image in "Air mould opacity": ∠ /*
  - *"Poor digestive aeration" image: / /*
  - *Other to be specified:*

- ***Hydrostatic and pneumatic washing:***
- *Lobster Claw image: / /*
- *"Cup-shaped stop" image: //*
- *Image in "Arret en trident": // o Other to be specified:*
- ***Abdominal scan:***

Abdominal mass: 1- Yes / / 2- No / /

- *Other a*

specify:

V. Treatment

1- Medical:

- *Analgesic: 1- Stage I / / 2- Stage II / 3- Stage III /_ /*
- *Antibiotherapy: 1- Mono /__ / 2- Bi /___ / 3- Tri /___ / 4- Other to be specified:*
- *Transfused: 1- Yes / / 2- No / /*

o Rehydration:

- *Hydrostatic reduction: 1- Yes / / 2- No / /*
- *Water reduction: 1- Yes / / 2- No / /*
- *Pneumatic reduction: 1- Yes / / 2- No / /*
- *Other to be specified:*

2- Surgical:

- *Simple manual reduction: 1- Yes / / 2- No / /*
- *End-to-end anastomosis resection: 1- Yes / / 2- No /___/*
- *Stoma: 1- Yes / / 2- No / /*
- *Other to be specified:*

3- Resuscitation:

- *Before surgery: 1- Yes / / 2- No / /*
- *After the operation: 1 - Yes // 2-No //*

VI. Evolution:

- *Favourable: 1- Yes / / 2- No //*
- *Complicated (s): 1- suppuration /_ /2- thread lachrymation // 3- eventration // 4- Evisceration // 5- Re-invagination // 6- Intestinal obstruction acute // 7- Post-operative peritonitis // 8- Other to be specified:*
- *Deceased: /___ /*

VII. Length of hospital stay:

In most cases, the after-effects are straightforward, with hospitalisation lasting between 02 and 21 days.

- *Cases in which reduction was surgical without resection required a hospital stay of between 02 days and 7 days.*
- *Cases whose reduction was surgical with resection required a hospital stay ranging from 03 days to 21 days.*
- *02 to 07 days: 1- Yes / / 2- No / /*

- ***08 to 15 days: 1- Yes /   / 2- No /   /***
- ***16 to 21 days: 1- Yes /   / 2- No /   /***
- ***More than 21 days: 1- Yes /   / 2- No /   /***

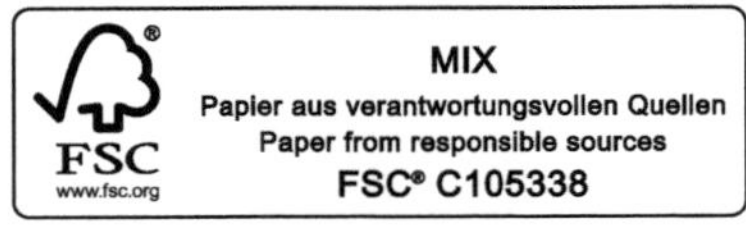

Printed by Books on Demand GmbH, Norderstedt / Germany